The ABC's of Good Nutrition

A Family's guide to Healthy Eating and Diet

For Children and Parents alike

By

Cheryl Powe

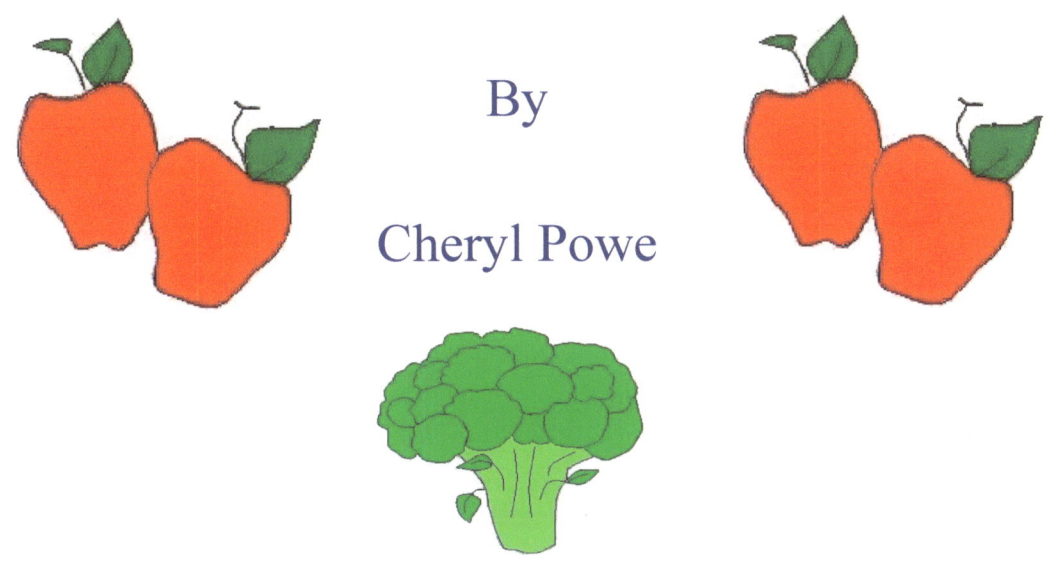

LCCN
All rights reserved
Copyright ©2015 by Cheryl Powe
CBK Publications Chicago, IL
Printed in the United States of America
ISBN 13: 978-1517264062

A

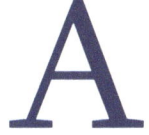

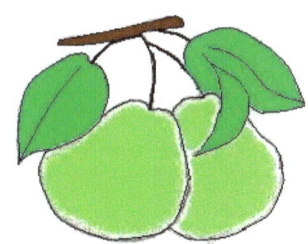

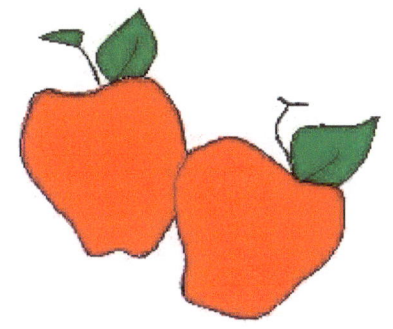

Apples and apricots, sweet and simple to eat. Whether they're for breakfast or lunch, they make a nice treat!

These fruits are healthy and good for the soul, they have all kinds of vitamins that help you to grow!

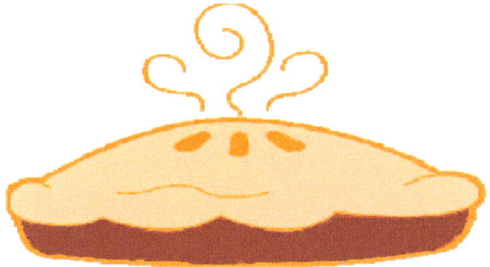

On Mondays, my mom loves to make us <u>homemade pies</u> and <u>fritters</u> made out of <u>apple and apricots</u>. She also makes caramel apples for dessert and after-school snacks.

My dad makes preserves with the fruits that he grows in our garden like peaches and grapes. We take the preserves and spread it on bread or pour some on our favorite dessert. It's very good and healthy for the body!

B

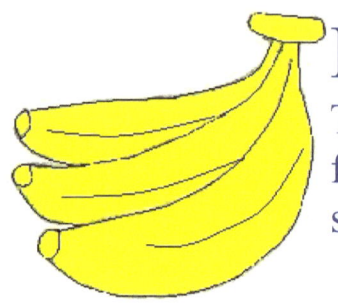

Bananas are yellow and mellow in taste. The   sweetness of the banana makes a happy face! When you are hungry, and in need of a snack, bananas are the best and that's a fact!

On Tuesdays, we love to eat bananas for breakfast. It can be used to make banana bread, banana waffles and sliced over cereal to give it that extra sweet taste, yummy!

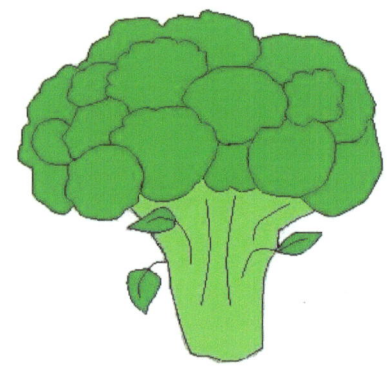

Broccoli

When we eat dinner, we use broccoli in our salads. We use it in dips with salad dressing. My mom also boils it, using seasonings and olive oil to substitute for butter as side a dish.

C

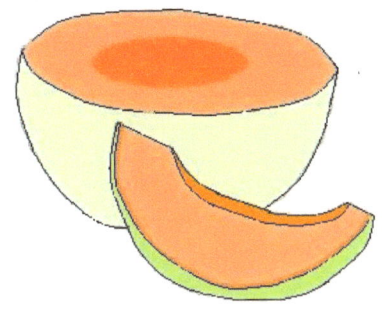

Cantaloupe is a melon and tastes very sweet. It can be served cool with its tasty juices, that's why it's good to eat!

On Wednesdays we eat cantaloupe because it is a sweet addition either by itself, in a fruit salad or in a smoothie. It all adds up to healthy yummy-ness!!

Corn and other vegetables are good to eat in soups; they're also good to eat raw, even in a group.

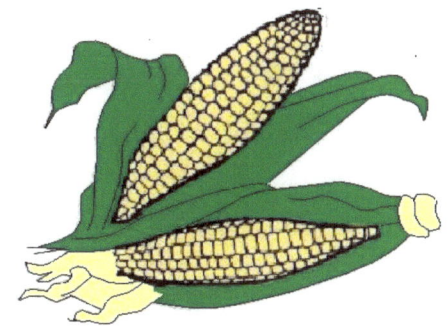

When we eat corn on the cob, my dad tells us to put a little bit of butter and some seasoning on it. My parents says you can either grill corn or fry it with pepper and onions on low heat in a skillet.

D

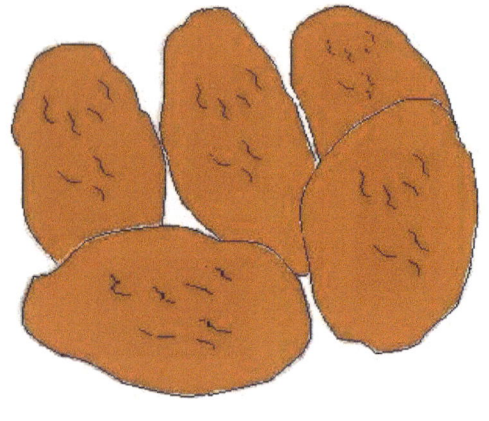

Dates look like raisins, but larger to hold; they are good to eat whether they're hot or cold!

On Thursdays, especially if it's around the holidays, mom and dad will bake pies and cakes. One of the cakes that they bake is a fruitcake. One of the fruits that goes into it are dates. Dates are so healthy to eat and when its put in a cake, that makes it fun and healthy to eat!

Dates can be used to make cookies, date bread and cereal bars. To find out recipes for this fruit, google recipes for dates on the internet.

E

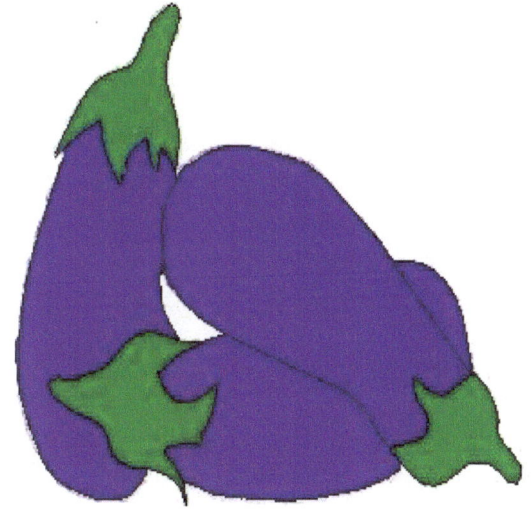

Eggplant is a vegetable that can be made into a meal such as, eggplant Parmesan and lasagna eggplant. It is a very healthy choice.

Then there's Friday when we have Eggplant Parmesan, which has spices and cheeses on it; lasagna eggplant has sauce, pasta and mozzarella cheese. Both are delicious and makes for a great dinner!

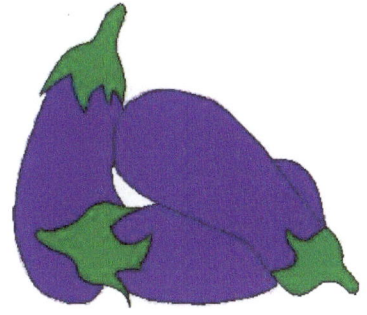

F

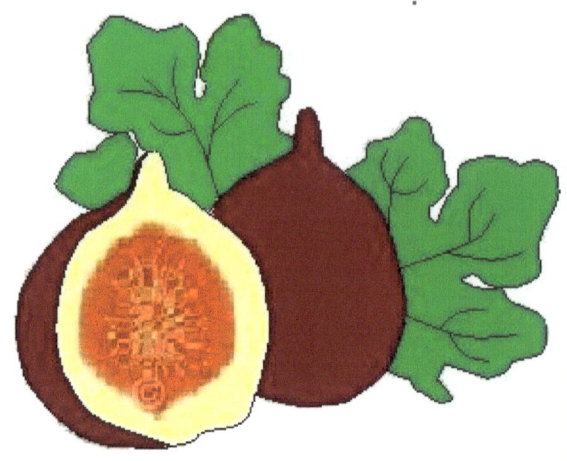

Figs are not dates and dates are not figs. Figs do not look like dates, but they're just as big.

Sometimes on Saturday and Sundays we might enjoy Figs which can be used in cakes, cookies, salads, pizza, in a preserve, a smoothie; and in a sauce for stuff leg of lamb. There are many recipes for figs and most of them can be found on the internet.

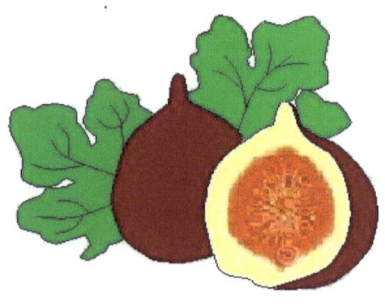

G

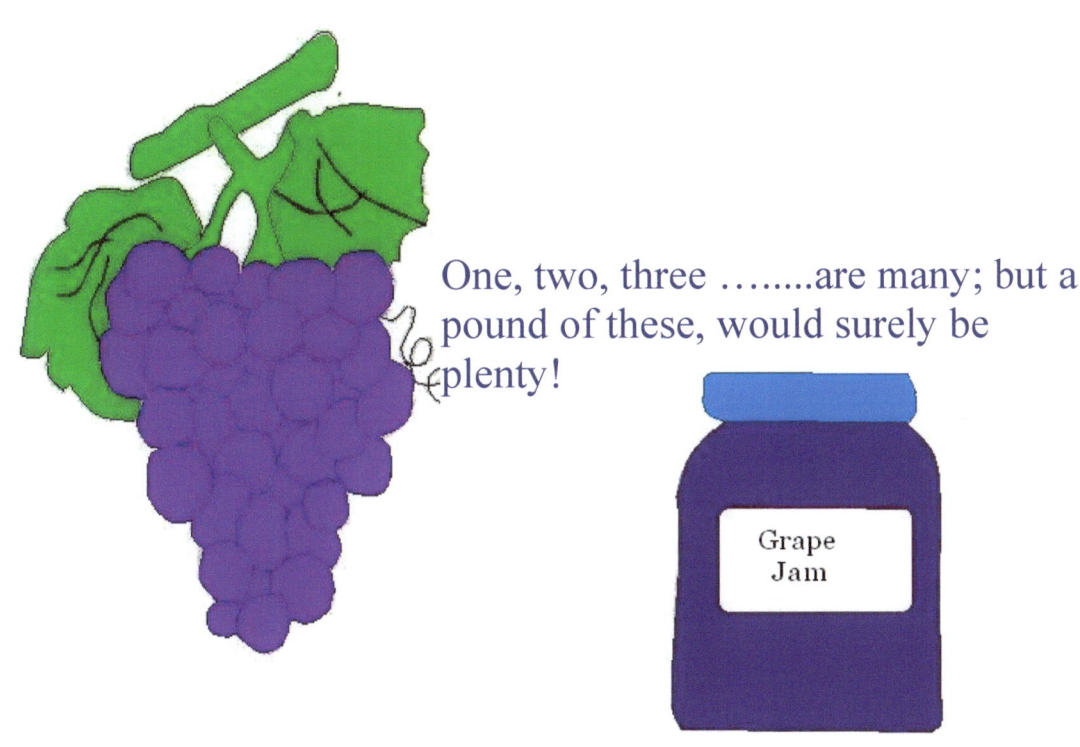

One, two, three ….......are many; but a pound of these, would surely be plenty!

Grape
Jam

Grapes make for a great snack to eat in between meals. They taste good, they're healthy and refreshing and makes for a great addition to a fruit salad.

Grapes can also be made into a freshly made jam or jelly that can be spreaded on toast, made as a peanut butter and jelly sandwich, and used as a filling for cakes. It can also be used on some meats such as pork chops and beefs. For more ideas and recipes, you can google "uses for grape jam" on the internet.

H

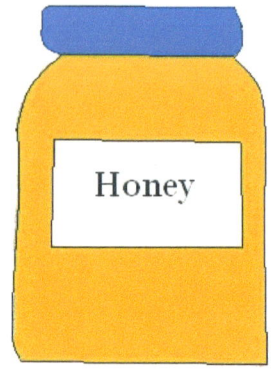

Honey is great and bees think so too; spread on toast, waffles and a variety of other stuff, through and through!

Raw honey is a great substitute for sugar. It carries all the natural ingredients that gives you energy to start the day. It can be used in salad dressing, in barbeque sauces, cakes, honey chicken wings, biscuits and cornbread too.

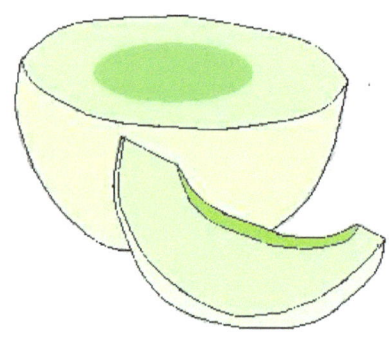

Honey Dew is the *cousin* to the cantaloupe because they look similar, except for the outer skin and color. Honey dews are sweet and juicy. They are very healthy to eat, enjoy and bon appetite!!

J

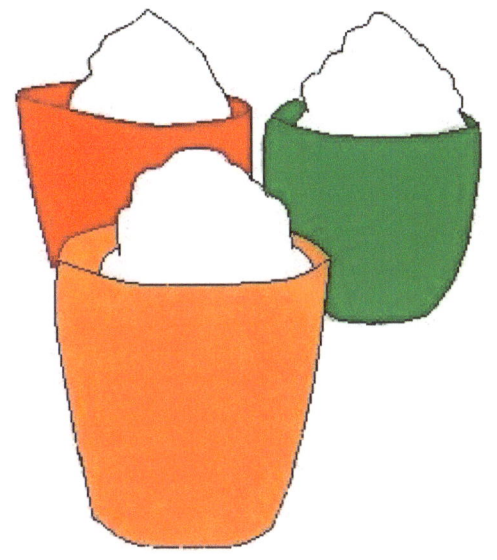

♫"I love <u>Jello</u>, I love jello......jello, jello, jello makes me kinda mellow!

Jello is a great snack and can be used as another choice to "junk food" that children eat. Be sure to get the ones that are low in sugar!

Recipes about jello for kids can be found on the internet at www.kraftrecipes.com

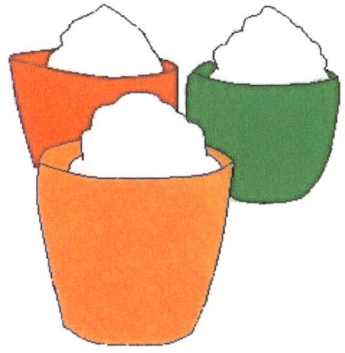

K

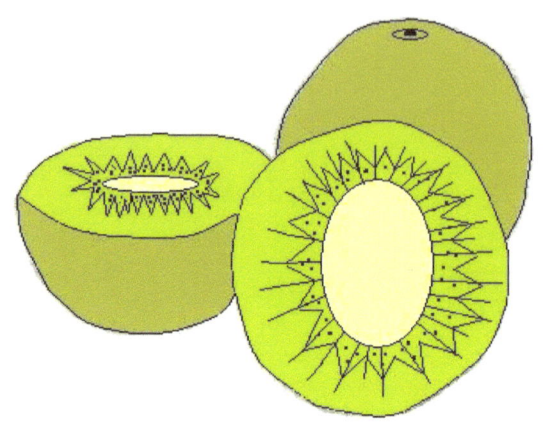

Kiwis are a small, sweet fruit that also has a tarty taste too! It's such a delight to eat and has many uses for recipes. We love kiwis!!

Kiwis can be used in fruit salads, fruitcakes, smoothies, baked in a fruit tart and in pizza *believe it or not!(fruity of course!)

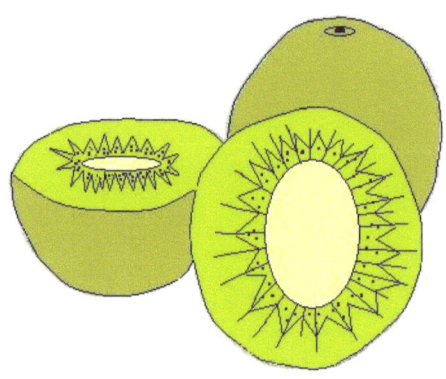

L

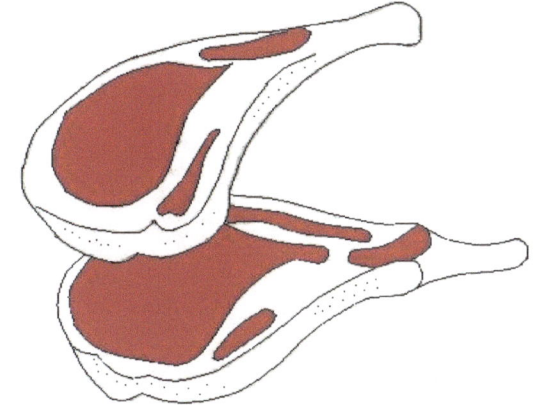

Lamb chops are not
pork chops, Pork chops comes
from a pig, lamb chops come
from the lamb and they're just as
big!!

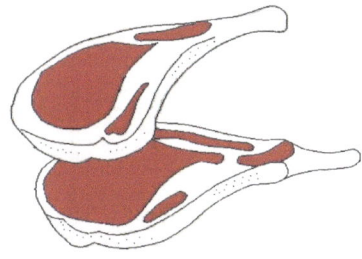

Lamb chops are best served baked, grilled or braised. Some of the
finer dishes that its served with is mash potatoes, rice; and
steamed vegetables such as broccoli, spinach, corn and broussel
sprouts....Yummy!!

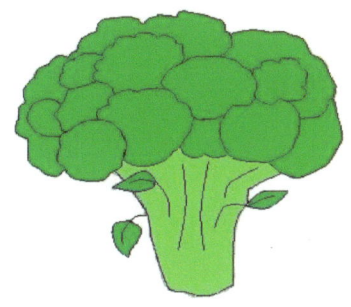

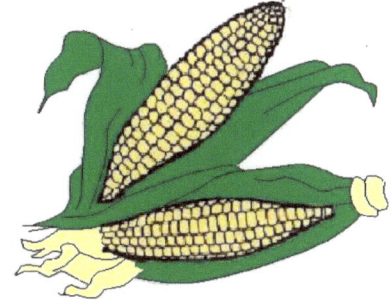

M

Milk builds a strong body and strong bones too!

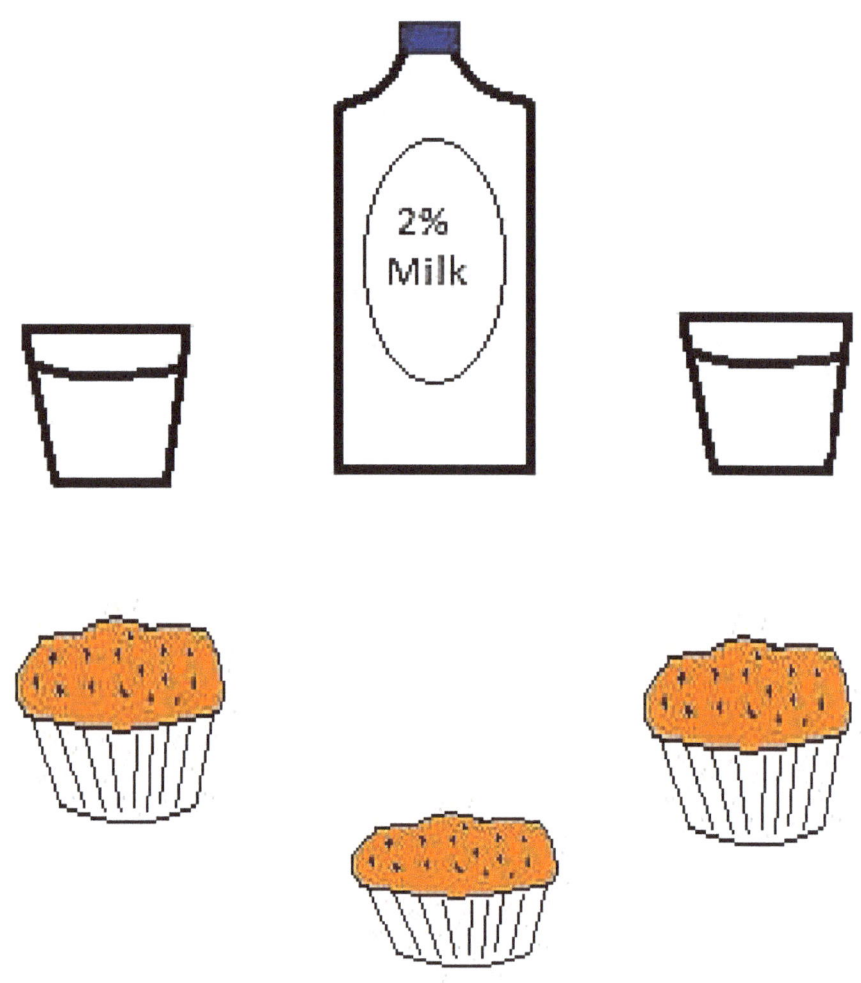

Muffins are a healthy treat and blueberry muffins are oh so sweet!!

N

Nectarines are small, like little balls of oranges. They're sweet and juicy and ripe with deliciousness!!

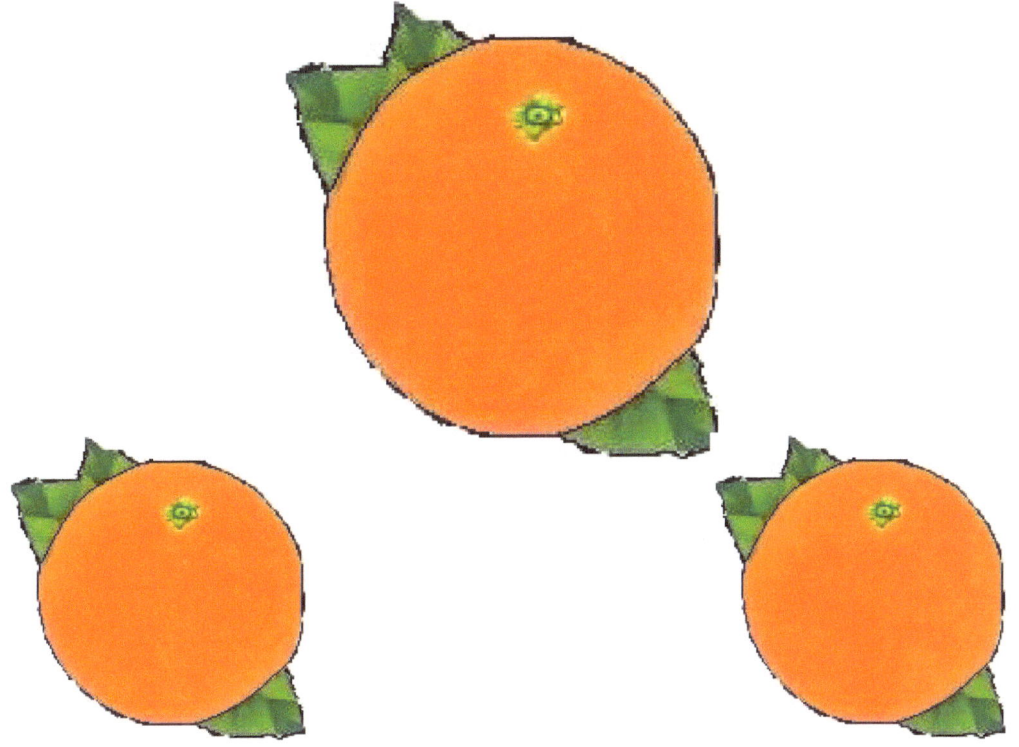

Nectarines can be used in smoothies, fruit salads or as an everyday snack. They're a nice and healthy snack for children to carry to school. Kids will love them!!

O

Oranges, oranges are a delicious treat.....like their cousin nectarines, they are so good to eat!!

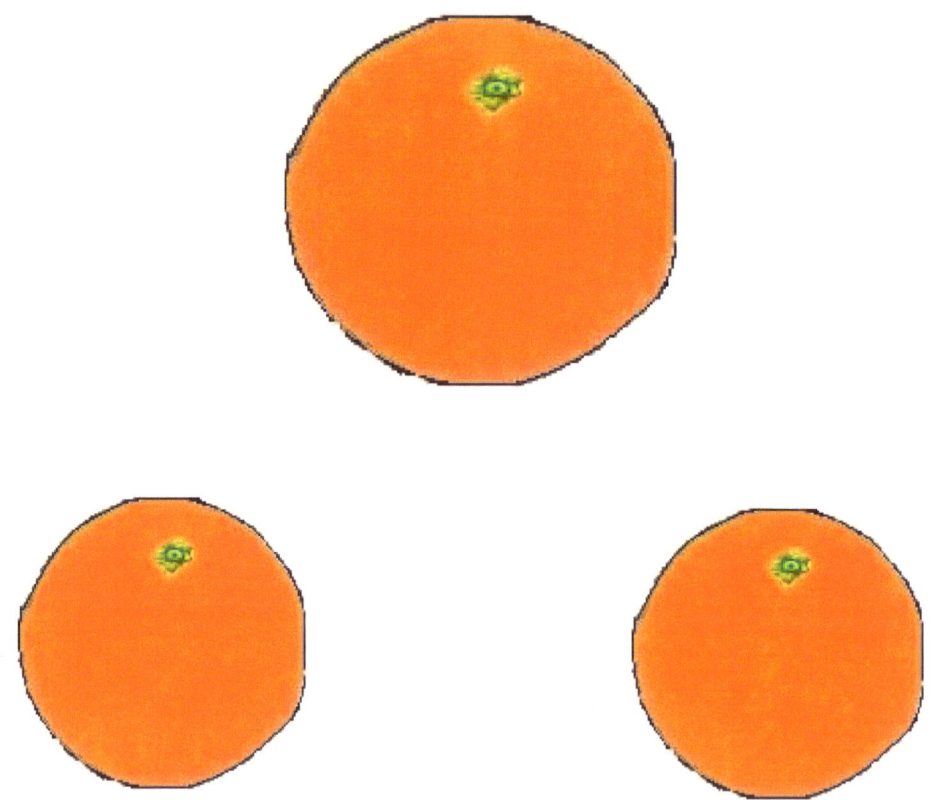

Oranges are squeeze to make orange juice, to put in fruit salads, orange flavoring in sherbert ice-cream and orange flavoring in cooking. It can also be put into cakes to make a delicious orange pound cake when baking.

P

When we think of **Pumpkins**, we think of the Autumn season.

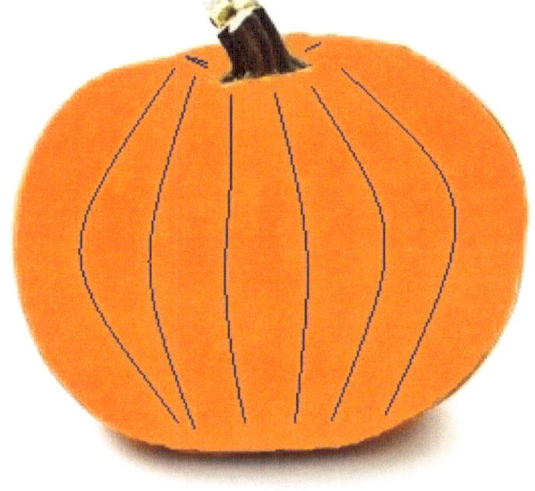

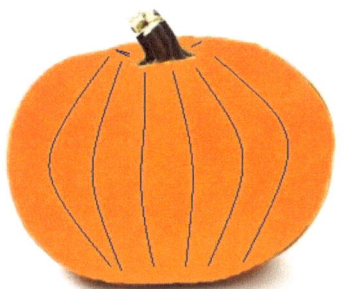 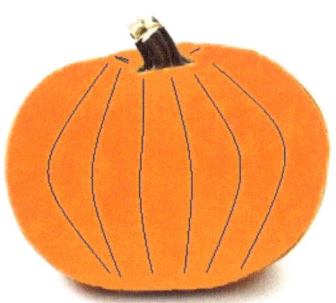

It seems like pumpkins are more plentiful during the Autumn time. The coolness of the fall brings delicious, plump pumpkins! Some people make pumpkin pies out of them, but my family usually make pumpkin seeds. You take the pumpkin seeds out of the pumpkin, rinse them off and spread on a sheet of foil paper.

Afterwards, you lightly sprinkle them with salt and bake in the oven. Cook to lightly brown and you have a wonderful healthy snack!!

R

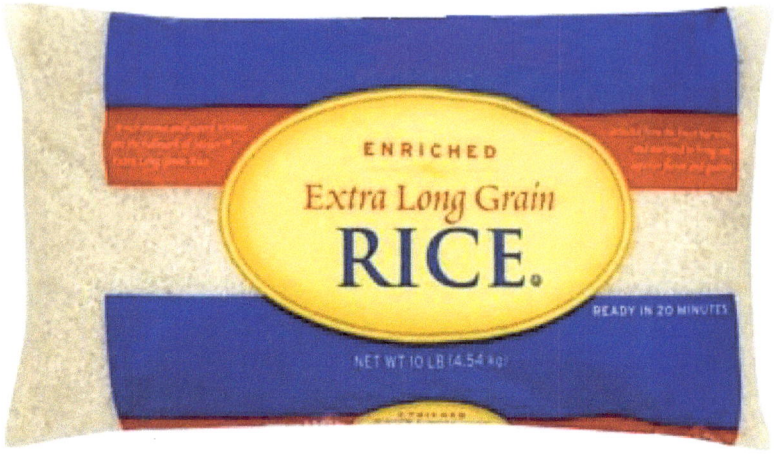

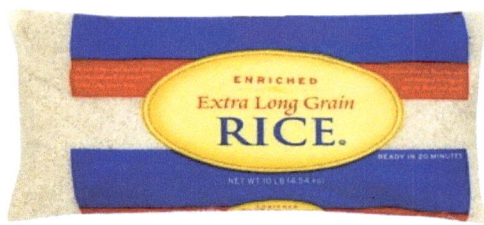

Rice is a favorite side dish for a lot of families. You can eat it with chicken, steak, lamb chops or even ground chuck. When it's cooked to the right kind of fluffiness, you can spread butter on it or top it off with gravy, it's great either way.

Rice can also be used as a dessert. You can make rice pudding out of it which makes for a healthy dessert for the entire family!! Google Rice pudding recipes to try it out!!

S

Strawberries

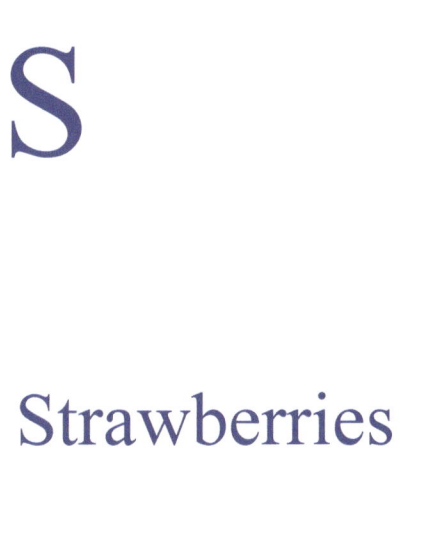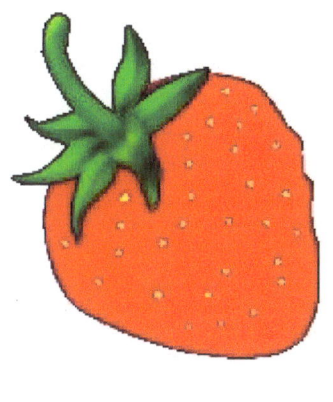

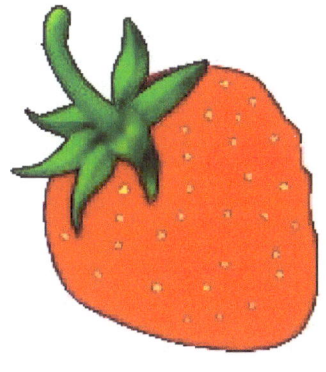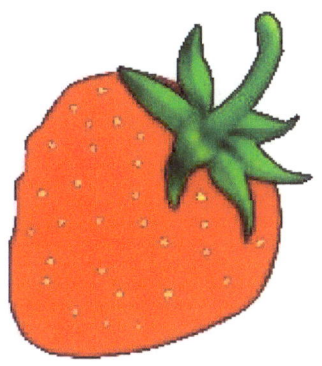

♫"Strawberries, get your fresh strawberries......come get your fresh strawberries right now!!♫

My family loves strawberries. You can eat strawberries as a snack, as a dessert and in a salad!! They are sweet and can be used in a strawberry shortcake. They are good and healthy for you!! Fresh Strawberries!!

T

Turkey

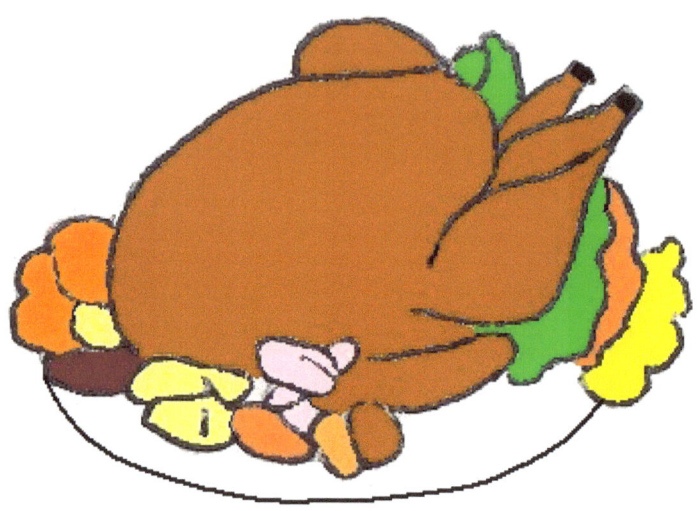

Turkey is very healthy and a nutritional meat for the entire family. It is less fat and more lean than most meats offered today!! Usually turkey is served during family dinners such as Thanksgiving and Christmas.

Leftover turkey can be used in soups, stews and also in sandwiches. Using turkey the day after it's been baked is usually a treat because all of the seasonings have simmered inside which makes for a delicious meal!!

W   Watermelon

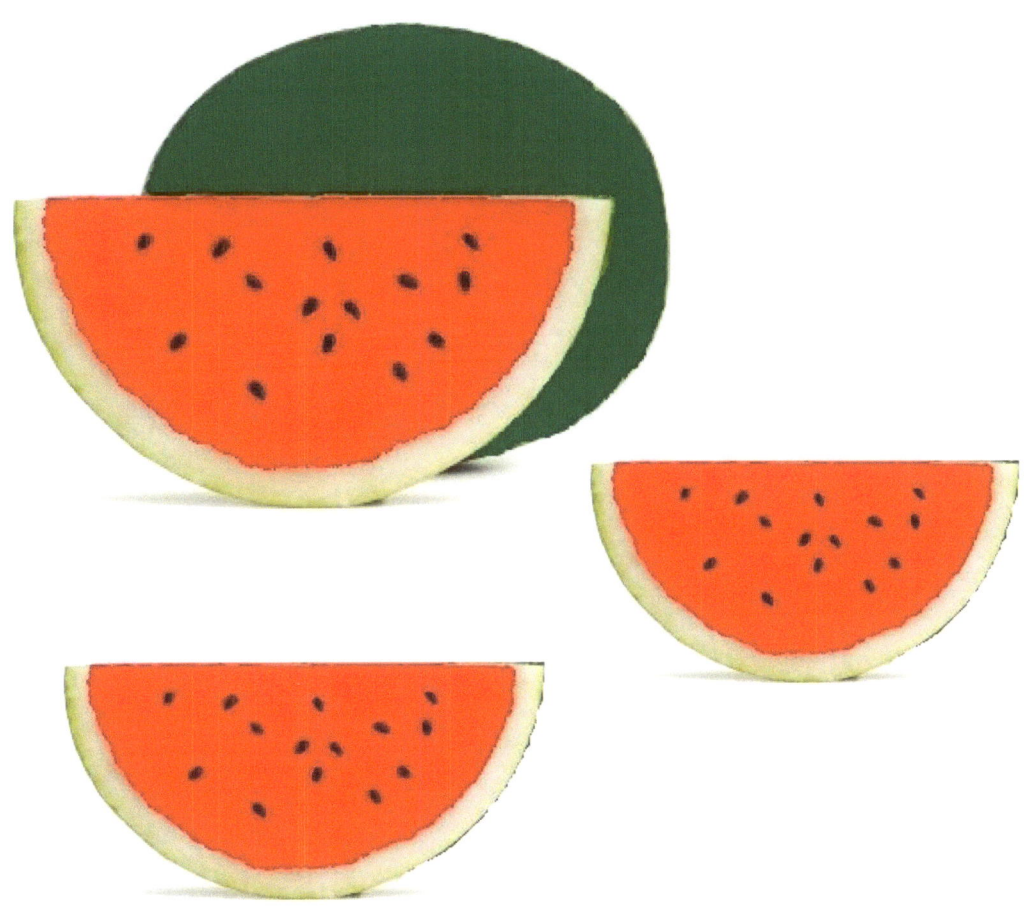

♫"Watermelon!!! Get your fresh, cold watermelon today"♫!!

Watermelon is a sweet, refreshing fruit, but most importantly its full of vitamins and nutrients that are good for your health! Watermelon contain lots of water that serves as a healthy fruit and good for your taste buds and soul!!

Y

Yams

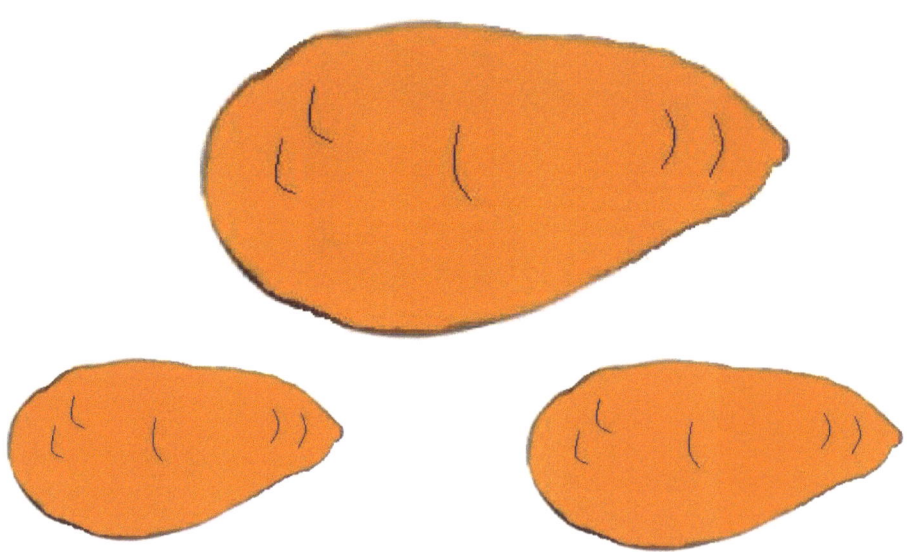

 Yams are another name for sweet potatoes.....and sweet potatoes are high in vitamins which means they're good for you!! Yams can be made into a pudding after you boil, mash and add sugar with flavor to them. You can also bake them with butter and sugar on them to make a nice treat!!

One of the most favorite things that you can do with the yam is make sweet potato pies with them. You can make it similar to the sweet potato pudding; afterwards pouring it into a floured pie shell, then baking it!! Makes for a delicious dessert!!

Z

Zucchini

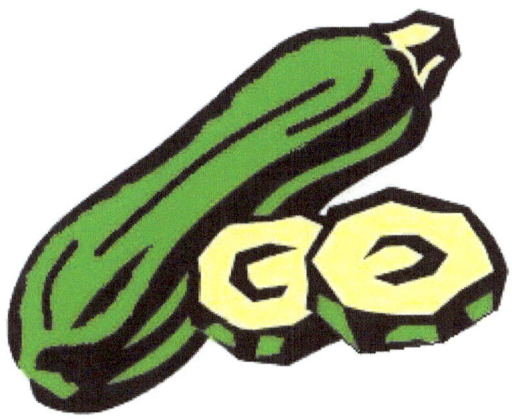

The Zucchini is a vegetable similar to the yellow squash only its green. It is a delicious vegetable that is so good when it is cut up, seasoned with garlic powder, season salt and pepper then grilled in olive oil.

It is the perfect side dish for fish, turkey, lambchops or chicken; and its a healthy way to get children started on their vegetables for the future!!

www.ingramcontent.com/pod-product-compliance
Lightning Source LLC
Chambersburg PA
CBHW060829290526
45792CB00005BB/1857